The Paleo Cast Iron Skillet

Disclaimer and Terms of Use:

Effort has been made to ensure that the information in this book is accurate and complete, however, the author and the publisher do not warrant the accuracy of the information, text and graphics contained within the book due to the rapidly changing nature of science, research, known and unknown facts and internet. The Author and the publisher do not hold any responsibility for errors, omissions or contrary interpretation of the subject matter herein. This book is presented solely for motivational and informational purposes only.

Table of Contents

Introduction

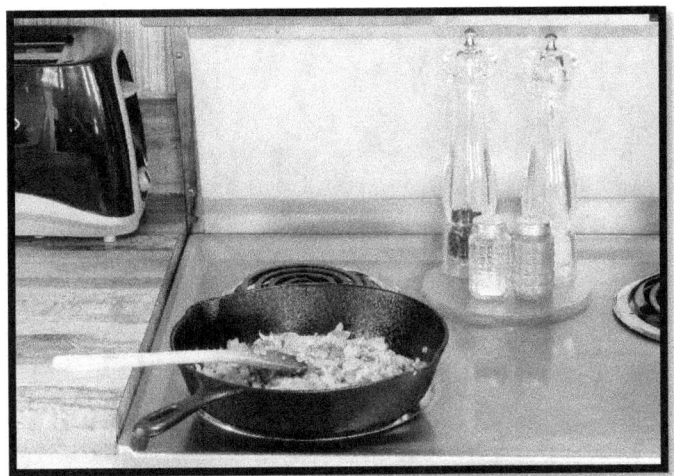

The Paleo diet is more than just another fad diet – it is a healthy lifestyle choice that countless individuals have turned to as a tool for improving their health. Many people assume that switching to the Paleo diet means that you have to give up your favorite foods. In reality, there are plenty of Paleo-friendly alternatives that allow you to keep making your favorite dishes. In this book you will find an assortment of Paleo cast iron skillet recipes which are not only full of flavor but very easy to make. With options like Sweet Potato Hash with Fried Eggs for breakfast and Blueberry Nectarine Cobbler for dessert, you won't feel like you are on a diet at all!

Paleo Cast Iron Recipes

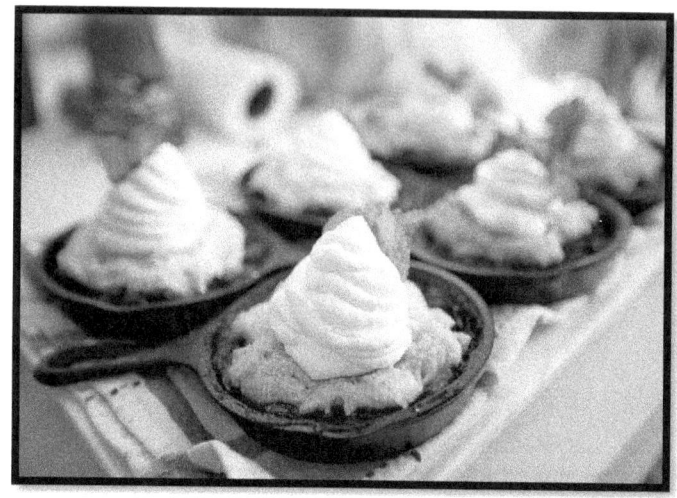

Recipes Included in this Book:

Skillet Eggs with Spinach

Sweet Potato Hash with Fried Eggs

Cinnamon Banana Pancakes

Lemon Blueberry Scones

Sausage Zucchini Skillet Frittata

Spicy Skillet Chili

Paleo Pizza with Veggies

Stir-Fried Cabbage and Mushrooms

Pan-Seared Steak over Mixed Greens

Pork and Sweet Potato Hash

Bacon-Wrapped Chicken Breasts

Southwestern-Style Shrimp Sauté

Herbed Pork Tenderloin

Chicken and Sausage Sauté

Cauliflower Pie with Meat Crust

Beef and Zucchini Stir-Fry

Coconut and Vegetable Curry

Pan-Seared Tilapia with Mango Salsa

Italian Chicken and Mushroom Skillet

Lemon Cherry Cake

Fudgy Chocolate Brownie

Pineapple Upside-Down Cake

Skillet Apple Crisp

Blueberry Nectarine Cobbler

Chocolate Chip Walnut Skillet Cookie

Skillet Eggs with Spinach

Servings: 4

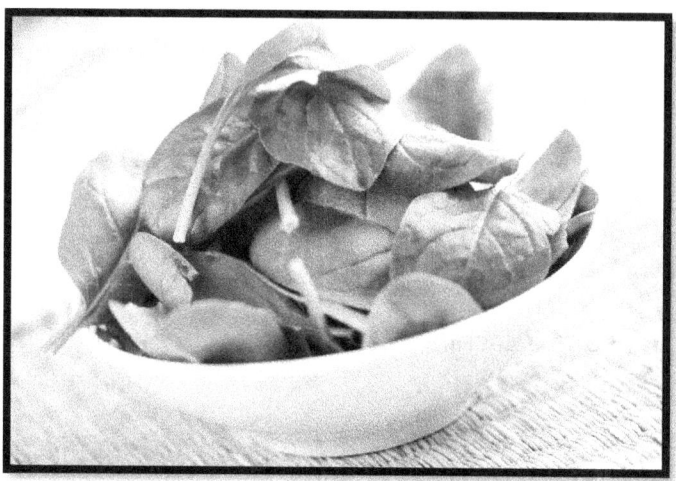

Ingredients:

6 to 8 slices uncooked bacon, chopped

6 ounces fresh baby spinach, chopped

4 large eggs

Salt and pepper to taste

Instructions:

1. Preheat the oven to 400°F.
2. Heat the bacon in a cast iron skillet over medium heat until crisp.
3. Remove the bacon to paper towel to drain and pour off the drippings.

4. Place the spinach in the skillet and season with salt and pepper to taste – cook for 1 minute until just wilted.
5. Stir in the bacon and spread the mixture evenly in the skillet.
6. Make four holes in the spinach mixture and crack an egg into each one.
7. Transfer the skillet to the oven and bake for 12 to 15 minutes until the eggs are set.
8. Season with salt and pepper to serve.

Sweet Potato Hash with Fried Eggs

Servings: 4

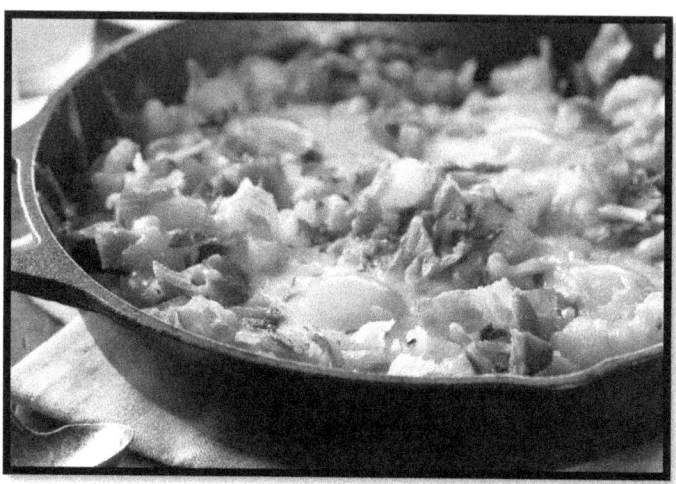

Ingredients:

4 medium sweet potatoes, peeled

¼ lbs. uncooked bacon, chopped

½ medium yellow onion, diced

4 large eggs

Salt and pepper to taste

Instructions:

1. Preheat the oven to 400°F.
2. Shred or finely chop the sweet potatoes and set them aside.
3. Heat the bacon in a cast iron skillet over medium-high heat.

4. Cook the bacon until crisp then remove it to paper towel to drain.
5. Add the sweet potatoes and onion to the skillet, stirring to coat with the bacon drippings.
6. Cook for 6 to 8 minutes, stirring often, until the sweet potato is tender.
7. Let the mixture cook for 2 to 3 minutes without disturbing until it forms a crust on the bottom.
8. Make four depressions in the sweet potato mixture and crack an egg into each.
9. Season the eggs with salt and pepper to taste.
10. Transfer the skillet to the oven and bake for 10 to 12 minutes until the eggs are set or until they are cooked to your liking.

Cinnamon Banana Pancakes

Servings: 4 to 6

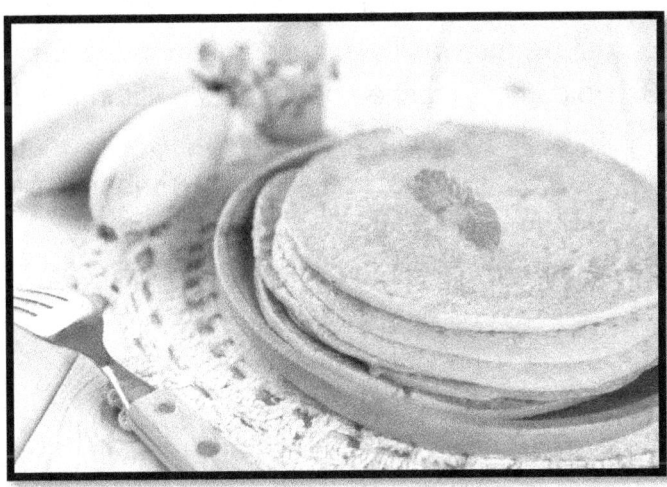

Ingredients:

1 ¼ cups almond flour

4 tablespoons coconut flour

¾ teaspoon baking soda

Pinch salt

1 cup canned coconut milk

3 large eggs

1 tablespoon maple syrup

1 teaspoon vanilla extract

1 large overripe banana, mashed

Instructions:

1. Sift together the almond flour, coconut flour, baking soda and salt into a large mixing bowl.
2. In a separate bowl, whisk together the coconut milk, eggs, vanilla extract, and maple syrup.
3. Fold in the mashed banana then stir in the dry ingredients until well combined.
4. Heat a large cast iron skillet over medium heat and grease with cooking oil.
5. Spoon the batter into the skillet using 2 to 3 tablespoons per pancake.
6. Cook the pancakes for 2 minutes or until bubbles form on the surface.
7. Carefully flip the pancakes and cook for 1 minute more or until lightly browned on the underside.

8. Transfer the pancakes to a plate to keep warm and repeat with the remaining batter.

Lemon Blueberry Scones

Servings: 8

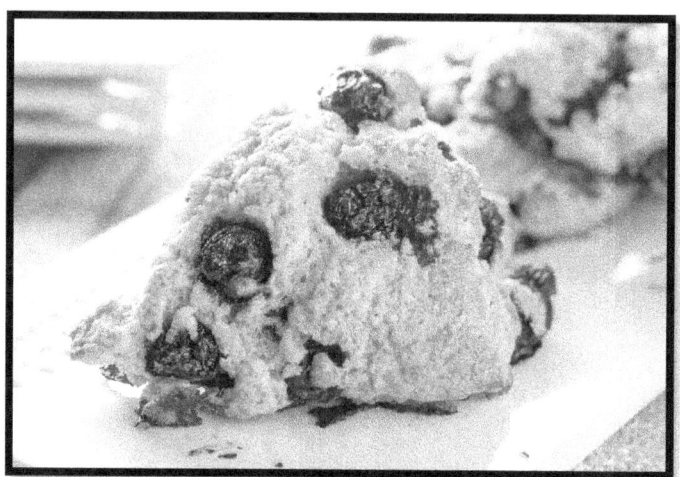

Ingredients:

1 ½ cups cashews, raw

½ cup tapioca flour

¾ teaspoon baking powder

Pinch salt

¼ cup fresh lemon juice

2 tablespoons unsweetened applesauce

1 ½ tablespoons coconut oil, melted

1 tablespoon almond milk, unsweetened

1 large egg

1 ½ teaspoons vanilla extract

1 cup fresh blueberries

1 tablespoon lemon zest

Instructions:

1. Preheat the oven to 350°F.
2. Place the cashews in a food processor and blend until they are finely ground.
3. Transfer the ground cashews to a mixing bowl and stir in the flour, baking powder, and salt.
4. In a separate bowl, whisk together the applesauce, coconut oil, almond milk, egg, vanilla extract, and lemon juice.
5. Stir the wet ingredients into the dry until smooth and well combined.
6. Fold in the blueberries and stir in the lemon zest.
7. Line a cast iron skillet with parchment paper and spread the batter in the skillet.
8. Place the skillet in the oven and bake for 25 to 30 minutes until a knife inserted in the center comes out clean.
9. Let the scones cool before slicing to serve.

Sausage Zucchini Skillet Frittata

Servings: 4 to 6

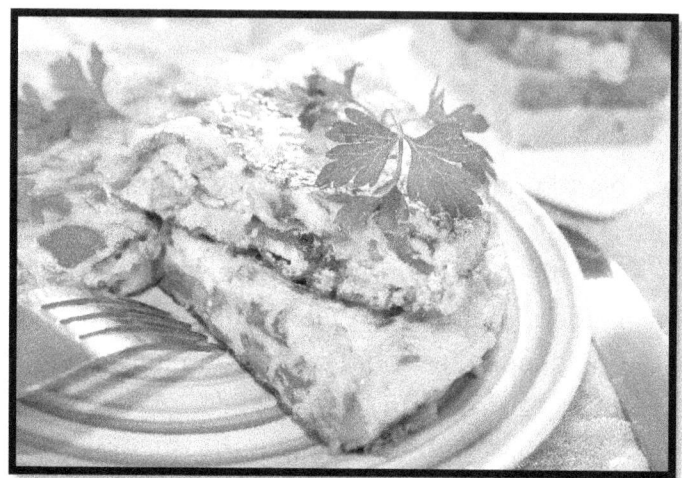

Ingredients:

10 large eggs

2 tablespoons unsweetened coconut milk

1 teaspoon salt

½ teaspoon black pepper

¼ lbs. ground pork sausage

2 small zucchini, finely diced

½ small red onion, sliced thin

½ red bell pepper, cored and chopped

Instructions:

1. Preheat the oven to 350°F.

2. Beat together the eggs, coconut milk, salt and pepper in a small bowl.
3. Heat the oil in a cast iron skillet over medium-high heat.
4. Add the sausage and cook for 2 to 3 minutes until evenly browned.
5. Stir in the zucchini, onion, and red pepper and cook for 4 to 5 minutes until just tender.
6. Pour the egg mixture into the cast iron skillet and stir well.
7. Transfer the skillet to the oven and bake for 20 to 25 minutes until the egg is set.
8. Cool the frittata for 3 to 5 minutes before slicing to serve.

Spicy Skillet Chili

Servings: 10 to 12

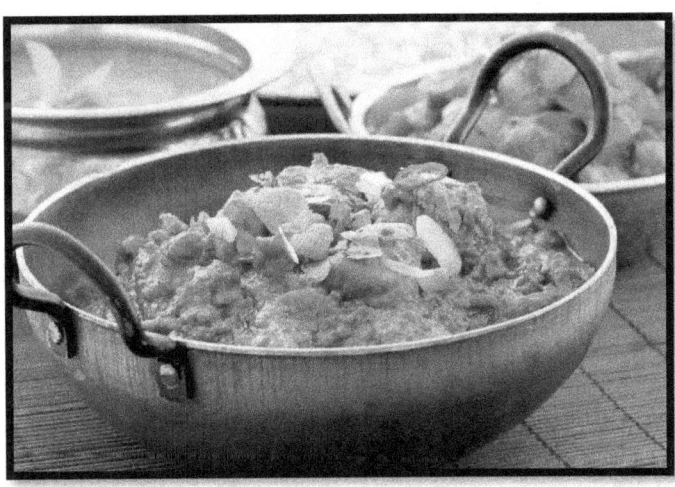

Ingredients:

3 tablespoons coconut oil

2 large sweet yellow onions, chopped

2 tablespoons minced garlic

2 lbs. lean ground beef

4 (14.5 ounce) cans diced tomatoes

2 cups beef stock

¼ cup chili powder

1 tablespoon dried oregano

1 teaspoon paprika

½ teaspoon ground cinnamon

2 tablespoons apple cider vinegar

Instructions:

1. Heat the oil in a large cast iron skillet over medium heat.
2. Stir in the onions and cook for 8 to 10 minutes until very soft.
3. Add the garlic and cook for 2 to 3 minutes.
4. Stir in the ground beef and cook for 5 to 6 minutes until evenly browned, breaking it into pieces with a wooden spoon as it cooks.
5. Add the tomatoes, beef stock, chili powder, oregano, and paprika.
6. Stir in the apple cider vinegar and cinnamon then reduce heat and simmer for 15 minutes.

7. Serve hot garnished with diced red onion.

Paleo Pizza with Veggies

Servings: 4

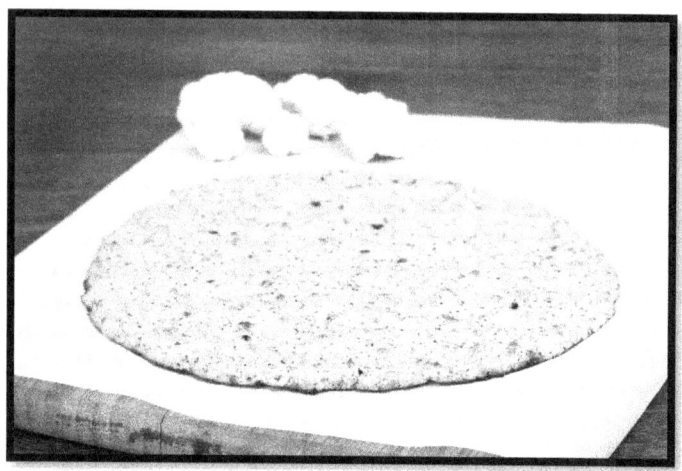

Ingredients:

1 cup cauliflower rice (cauliflower florets chopped in food processor)

1 large egg

1 teaspoon garlic powder

½ teaspoon dried oregano

Pinch salt

¼ cup tomato sauce

2 cups assorted sliced veggies

Instructions:

1. Preheat the oven to 450°F.

2. Combine the cauliflower, egg, garlic powder, oregano and salt in a mixing bowl.
3. Stir the ingredients until well combined then pack the mixture into a small greased cast iron skillet, pressing it into the bottom and sides like a pie crust.
4. Bake the crust for 12 to 15 minutes.
5. Remove the skillet from the oven and top the crust with tomato sauce and sprinkle with vegetables.
6. Return the skillet to the oven for 5 to 8 minutes until the vegetables are hot.
7. Slice the pizza to serve.

Stir-Fried Cabbage and Mushrooms

Servings: 4

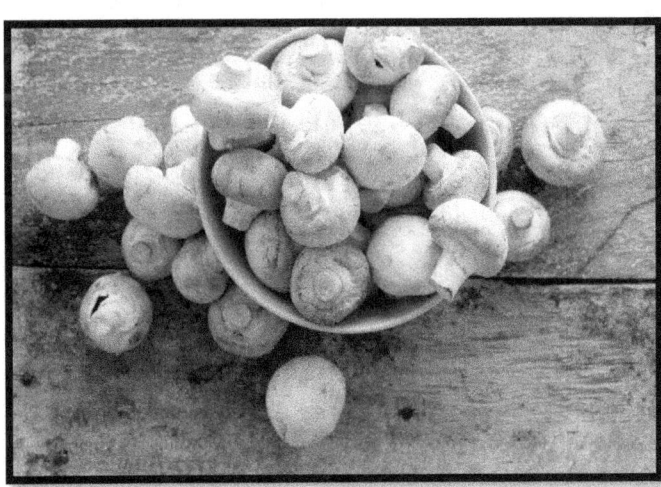

Ingredients:

1 tablespoon coconut oil

4 slices uncooked bacon, chopped

2 medium leeks, sliced (white and light green parts)

Salt and pepper to taste

½ cup chicken broth, divided

6 cups savoy cabbage, sliced thin

8 ounces sliced mushrooms

Instructions:

1. Heat the oil in a large cast iron skillet over low heat.
2. Add the bacon and cook for 4 to 5 minutes until crisp then transfer to paper towels to drain.
3. Reheat the skillet then stir in the leeks – season with salt and pepper to taste.
4. Add ¼ cup chicken broth then simmer the mixture for 5 minutes until the leeks are tender.
5. Stir in the cabbage and the remaining chicken broth then cover and simmer for 12 to 15 minutes until very tender.
6. Add the mushrooms then simmer for 5 to 6 minutes more.
7. Sprinkle with the chopped bacon to serve.

Pan-Seared Steak over Mixed Greens

Servings: 6

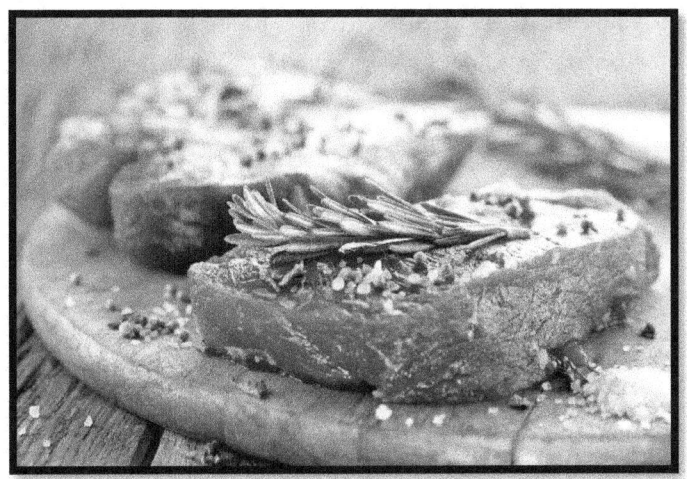

Ingredients:

1 ½ lbs. flank steak

Salt and pepper to taste

1 tablespoon olive oil

6 cups mixed spring greens

Instructions:

1. Season the steak liberally with salt and pepper to taste.
2. Heat the oil in a large cast iron skillet over high heat.
3. Add the steaks and cook for 4 minutes then flip the steaks and cook for another 3 to 5 minutes until cooked to the desired level.
4. Remove the steaks to a cutting board and let rest for 5 minutes before slicing thin.

5. Divide the greens among four plates and top with the sliced steak to serve.

Pork and Sweet Potato Hash

Servings: 4

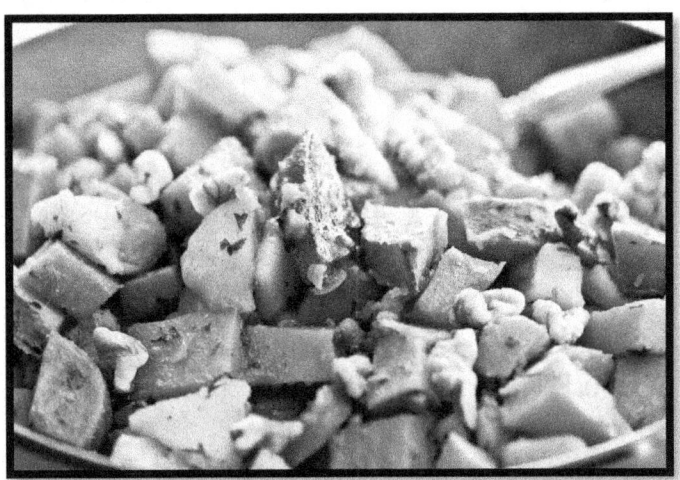

Ingredients:

1 lbs. ground pork

2 tablespoons minced garlic

3 cups chicken broth

4 cups diced sweet potato

1 cup diced yellow onion

1 cup diced cauliflower florets

Salt and pepper to taste

1 teaspoon chili powder

2 green onions, sliced thin

Instructions:

1. Heat the pork in a large cast iron skillet over medium-high heat.
2. Cook for 7 to 8 minutes, stirring often, until the pork is evenly browned.
3. Stir in the garlic and chicken broth then bring the mixture to a boil.
4. Add the sweet potato, onion, and cauliflower.
5. Season the mixture with salt and pepper to taste then stir in the chili powder.
6. Reduce heat and simmer for 15 to 20 minutes until the vegetables are tender.
7. Sprinkle with green onions to serve.

Bacon-Wrapped Chicken Breasts

Servings: 4

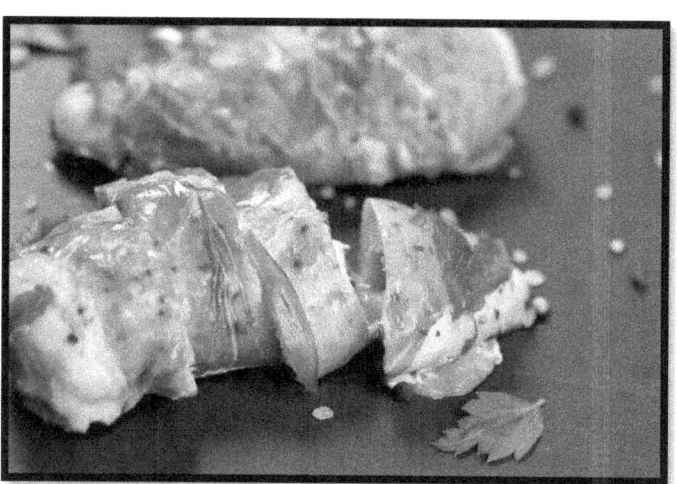

Ingredients:

1 tablespoon olive oil

2 teaspoons minced garlic

2 tablespoons fresh chopped rosemary

2 tablespoons fresh lemon juice

1 teaspoon dried thyme

4 (4 to 6 ounce) boneless skinless chicken breasts

6 to 8 slices uncooked bacon

Instructions:

1. Combine the olive oil, garlic, rosemary, lemon juice and thyme in a freezer bag.
2. Add the chicken and toss to coat then chill for at least 1 hour up to 8 hours.
3. Remove the chicken breasts from the bag and wrap each in one or two slices of bacon – use wooden toothpicks to secure the slices.
4. Heat the coconut oil in a large cast iron skillet over medium heat.
5. Add the chicken breasts and cook for 8 to 10 minutes per side until the chicken is cooked through and the bacon crisp.
6. Remove the chicken to a cutting board and let rest for 5 minutes before slicing to serve.

Southwestern-Style Shrimp Sauté

Servings: 4

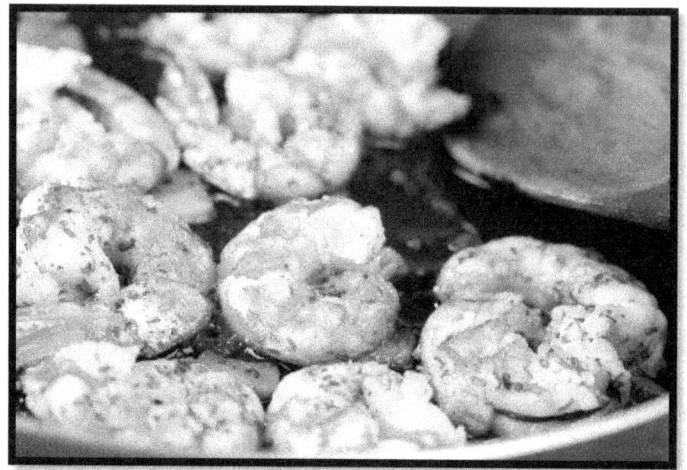

Ingredients:

2 tablespoons olive oil

2 medium red onions, diced

6 small stalks celery, diced

2 large ripe tomatoes, cored and chopped

2 red bell peppers, cored and chopped

1 ½ lbs. uncooked shrimp, peeled and deveined

Chipotle chili powder to taste

Instructions:

1. Preheat the oven to 400°F.
2. Heat the oil in a large cast iron skillet over medium heat.
3. Add the onions and cook for 4 to 5 minutes until they are translucent.

4. Stir in the celery, tomatoes, and red peppers and cook for 8 to 10 minutes.
5. Add the shrimp and sprinkle with chipotle chili powder.
6. Cook for 2 to 3 minutes until the shrimp just turns pink.
7. Serve the shrimp hot over cauliflower rice or steamed spaghetti squash.

Beef and Zucchini Stir-Fry

Servings: 4

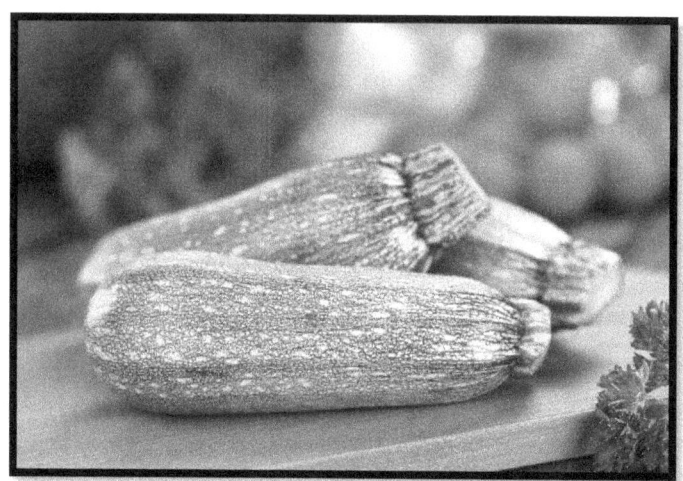

Ingredients:

1 tablespoon coconut oil

1 large yellow onion, sliced thin

1 medium red pepper, cored and sliced

1 lbs. ground beef

3 cups chopped zucchini

1 (14 ounce) can chopped tomatoes

½ cup beef broth

1 tablespoon chili powder

Salt and pepper to taste

Instructions:

1. Heat the oil in a large cast iron skillet over medium-high heat.
2. Add the onion and bell peppers then sauté for 5 to 6 minutes until tender.
3. Stir in the ground beef and cook for 3 to 4 minutes until evenly browned.
4. Add the zucchini, tomatoes, and beef broth then stir well.
5. Stir in the chili powder, salt and pepper then cover the skillet and simmer for 15 minutes until the vegetables are tender and the beef is cooked through.
6. Serve the stir-fry hot over cauliflower rice.

Herbed Pork Tenderloin

Servings: 6

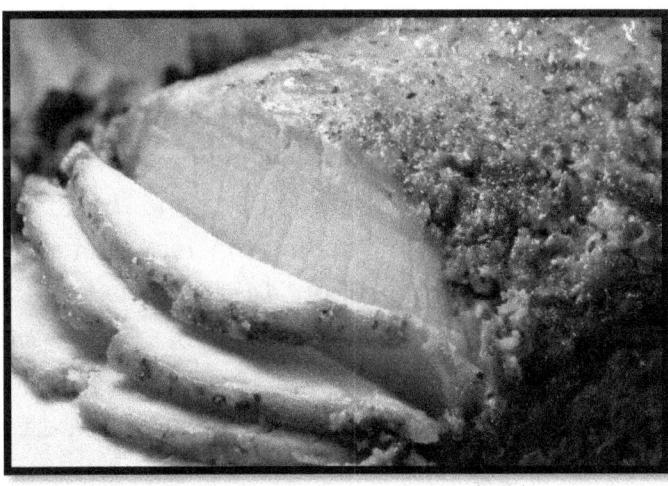

Ingredients:

2 (1 ½ to 2 lbs.) boneless pork tenderloins

1 tablespoons dried parsley

½ tablespoon dried rosemary

1 teaspoon dried oregano

½ teaspoon dried thyme

Salt and pepper to taste

2 tablespoons coconut oil

Instructions:

1. Preheat the oven to 425°F.
2. Trim the extra fat from the tenderloins and pat it dry with paper towel.
3. Combine the spices in a small bowl and season with salt and pepper to taste – rub the mixture into the pork on all sides.
4. Heat the oil in a cast iron skillet over medium heat.
5. Add the pork tenderloins and cook for 2 minutes on each side until evenly browned.
6. Transfer the skillet to the oven and roast for 12 to 15 minutes until the internal temperature of each tenderloin is about 145°F.
7. Remove the pork to a cutting board and cover loosely with foil.
8. Let rest for 10 minutes before slicing to serve.

Chicken and Sausage Sauté

Servings: 6

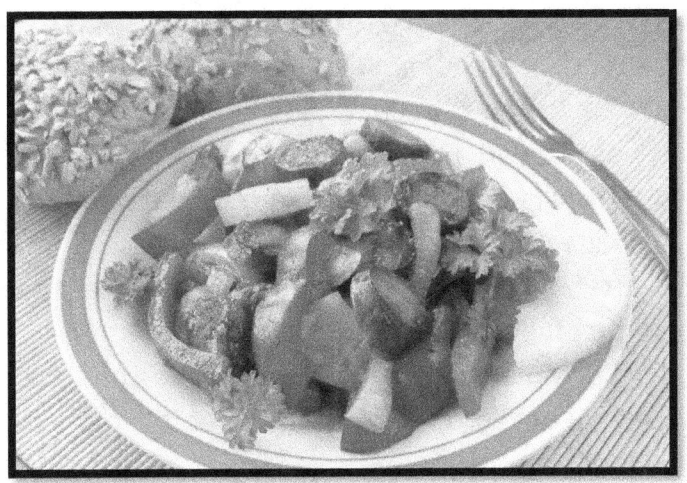

Ingredients:

1 ½ lbs. chicken thighs and drumsticks

Salt and pepper to taste

2 tablespoons coconut oil

½ lbs. Italian sausage links

1 medium yellow onion, sliced

1 red bell pepper, cored and sliced

1 yellow bell pepper, cored and sliced

½ cup chicken broth

Instructions:

1. Season the chicken with salt and pepper to taste then set aside.

2. Heat the oil in a large cast iron skillet over medium heat then add the sausage.
3. Cook the sausage for 6 to 7 minutes, turning as needed, until evenly browned.
4. Transfer the sausage to a cutting board and slice it.
5. Reheat the skillet over medium-high heat and add the chicken.
6. Cook the chicken for 2 to 3 minutes on each side until browned then transfer to a plate to keep warm.
7. Add the onion, red pepper and yellow peppers to the skillet and cook for 4 to 5 minutes until tender-crisp.
8. Return the chicken and sausage to the pan and pour in the chicken broth.
9. Cover and simmer the mixture on low heat for 15 to 20 minutes until the chicken is cooked through.

Cauliflower Pie with Meat Crust

Servings: 6 to 8

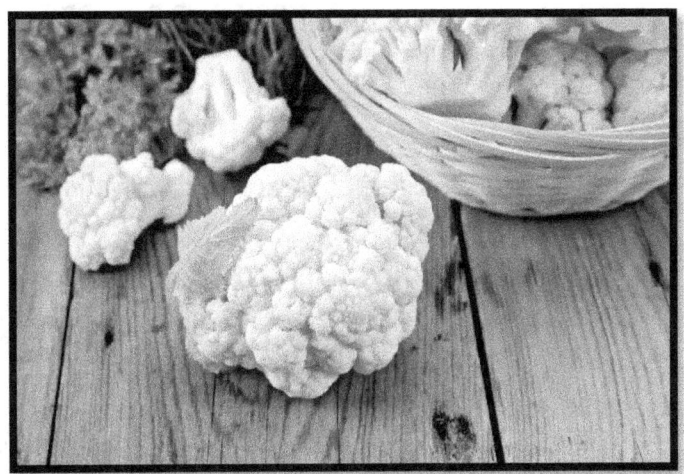

Ingredients:

2 medium heads cauliflower, chopped

10 cloves garlic, minced

¼ cup extra-virgin olive oil

2 lbs. lean ground beef

2 tablespoons ground flaxseed

1/3 cup water

1 tablespoon garlic powder

½ tablespoon onion powder

4 slices cooked bacon, crumbled

1 green onion, sliced thin

Instructions:

1. Preheat the oven to 375°F.
2. Spread the cauliflower and garlic on a rimmed baking sheet and toss with olive oil.
3. Roast the cauliflower for 30 minutes, turning once.
4. Whisk together the flaxseed and water in a small bowl and let rest 5 minutes.
5. Combine the ground beef, garlic powder, and onion powder with the flax mixture in a mixing bowl.
6. Spread the meat mixture in a medium cast iron skillet, pressing it into the bottom and sides like a pie crust.
7. Bake the crust for 15 minutes.
8. Combine the roasted cauliflower and garlic in a food processor and blend smooth.
9. Spread the cauliflower puree in the meat crust and top with crumbled bacon and sliced green onion.
10. Bake for 15 minutes or until the top of the pie is lightly browned.

Coconut and Vegetable Curry

Servings: 4 to 6

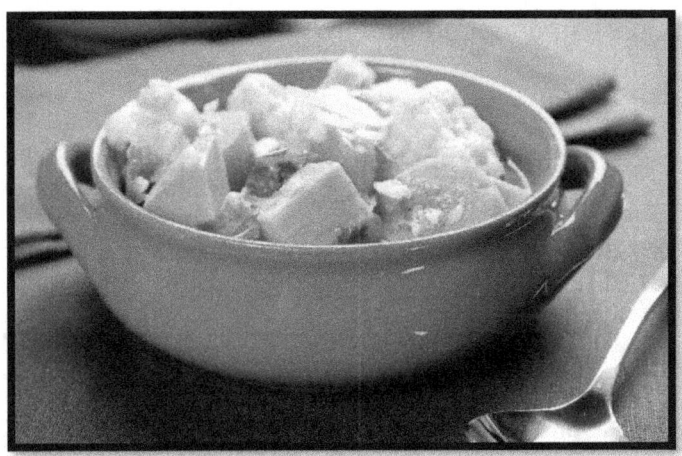

Ingredients:

1 tablespoon coconut oil

1 tablespoon fresh minced garlic

1 tablespoon fresh grated ginger

1 medium yellow onion, chopped

1 cup chopped carrots

2 cups chopped cauliflower florets

1 tablespoon curry powder

1 cup vegetable broth

2 (14 ounce) cans coconut milk

Salt and pepper to taste

½ cup diced tomatoes

½ cup snow peas

¼ cup fresh chopped cilantro

Instructions:

1. Heat 1 tablespoon coconut oil in a large cast iron skillet over medium heat.
2. Add the garlic and ginger and cook for 1 minute.
3. Stir in the onion, carrots, and cauliflower then season with salt and pepper to taste.
4. Cook for 4 to 5 minutes until the onion is softened.
5. Stir in the curry powder, vegetable broth, and coconut milk then season with salt and pepper again.
6. Cook for 12 to 15 minutes until the vegetables are very tender.
7. Stir in the tomatoes, snow peas and cilantro during the last 5 minutes of cooking.
8. Serve the curry hot over cauliflower rice.

Pan-Seared Tilapia with Mango Salsa

Servings: 4

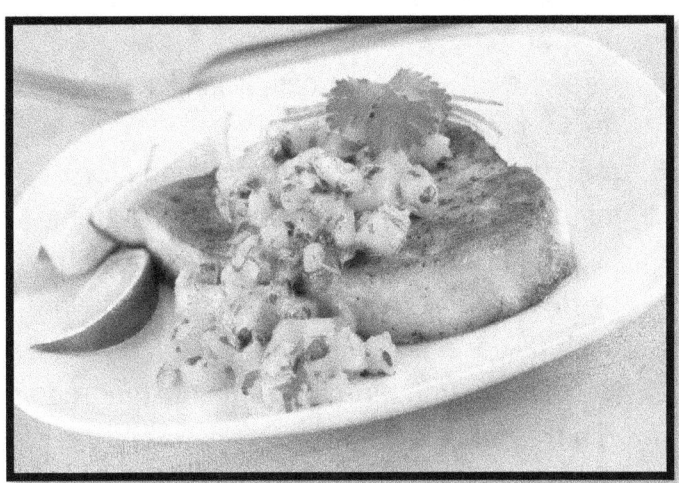

Ingredients:

4 (6 ounce) tilapia fillets

2 tablespoons olive oil

Salt and pepper to taste

1 large ripe mango, pitted and finely diced

2 tablespoons diced red onion

2 tablespoons fresh chopped cilantro

1 tablespoon fresh lime juice

Instructions:

1. Preheat the oven to 300°F.

2. Rinse the fillets with cool water then pat dry with paper towel.
3. Generously season the fillets with salt and pepper to taste.
4. Heat the oil in a large cast iron skillet over medium heat until very hot.
5. Add the fillets to the skillet and cook for 5 minutes until golden brown on the bottom.
6. Flip the fillets then transfer the skillet to the oven and cook for 5 minutes or so until the flesh flakes easily with a fork.
7. Meanwhile, combine the remaining ingredients in a mixing bowl.
8. Serve the fillets hot topped with the mango salsa.

Italian Chicken and Mushroom Skillet

Servings: 4

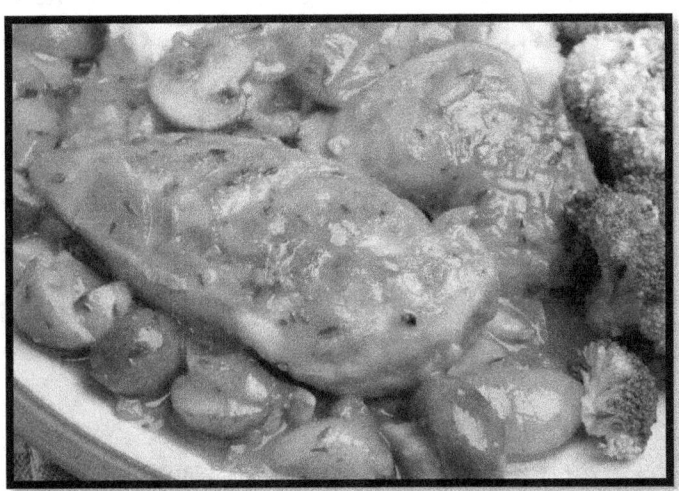

Ingredients:

2 tablespoons coconut oil, divided

1 lbs. boneless skinless chicken breast tenderloins

12 ounces sliced mushrooms

1 medium yellow onion, chopped

1 tablespoon minced garlic

½ cup sun-dried tomatoes in oil, drained and chopped

1 teaspoon dried oregano

Salt and pepper to taste

Instructions:

1. Heat 1 tablespoon coconut oil in a large cast iron skillet over medium-high heat.
2. Add the chicken and cook for 2 to 3 minutes on each side until browned.
3. Remove the chicken to a plate to keep warm and reheat the skillet with another tablespoon of oil.
4. Add the mushrooms and cook for 2 to 3 minutes then flip them and cook for another 2 to 3 minutes until browned.
5. Stir in the onion, garlic, and sun-dried tomatoes and cook for 5 minutes until the onion is tender.
6. Add the oregano and season with salt and pepper to taste.
7. Return the chicken to the pan then cover the skillet and cook for 10 to 12 minutes until the chicken is cooked through.

Lemon Cherry Cake

Servings: 6 to 8

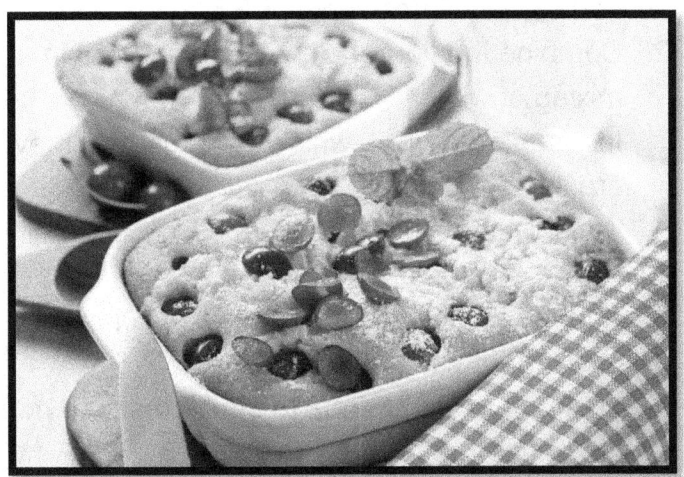

Ingredients:

½ cup sifted coconut flour

¾ teaspoon baking soda

Pinch salt

6 large eggs, beaten

1/3 cup raw honey

½ cup coconut oil, melted

1/3 cup canned coconut milk

1 ½ tablespoons fresh lemon juice

1 teaspoon vanilla extract

1 cup fresh cherries, pitted and halved

Instructions:

1. Preheat the oven to 350°F and grease a cast iron skillet with cooking oil.
2. Combine the flour, baking soda and salt in a mixing bowl.
3. In a separate bowl, whisk the eggs until they are light and foamy.
4. Whisk in the honey, coconut oil, coconut milk, vanilla extract, and lemon juice.
5. Add the dry ingredients to the wet, whisking until smooth and well combined.
6. Let the mixture sit for 2 to 3 minutes then pour the batter into the skillet.
7. Sprinkle the cherries over the batter and bake for 26 to 30 minutes until a knife inserted in the center comes out clean.

Fudgy Chocolate Brownie

Servings: 4

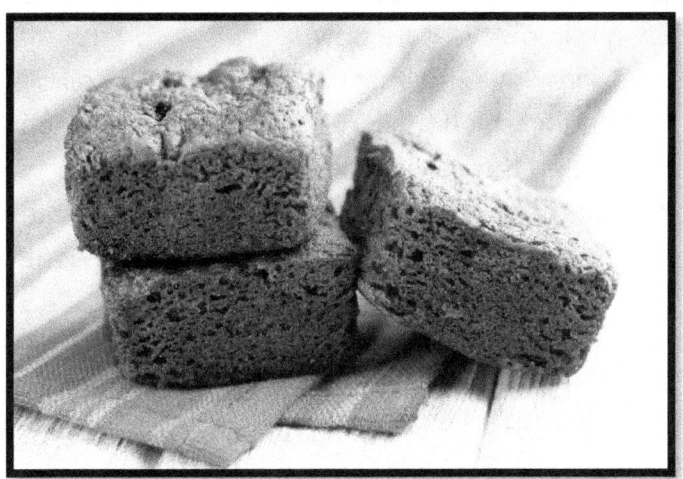

Ingredients:

¼ cup coconut oil

1 cup dark chocolate chips (at least 65% cacao)

½ small overripe banana, mashed

1 teaspoon vanilla extract

Pinch salt

2 large eggs, beaten

1/3 cup tapioca flour

½ tablespoon coconut flour

Instructions:

1. Preheat the oven to 350°F and grease a small cast iron skillet with oil.
2. Combine the coconut oil and dark chocolate in a microwave-safe bowl.
3. Microwave the chocolate and coconut oil on medium-high heat in 15-second intervals until melted then stir smooth.
4. Stir the banana, vanilla extract, and salt into the melted chocolate then whisk in the eggs one at a time.
5. Whisk in the flours until smooth and well combined then spread the batter in the skillet.
6. Bake for 20 to 22 minutes until the edges of the brownie are crisp and start to pull away from the sides.
7. Cool the brownie completely before serving.

Pineapple Upside-Down Cake

Servings: 6 to 8

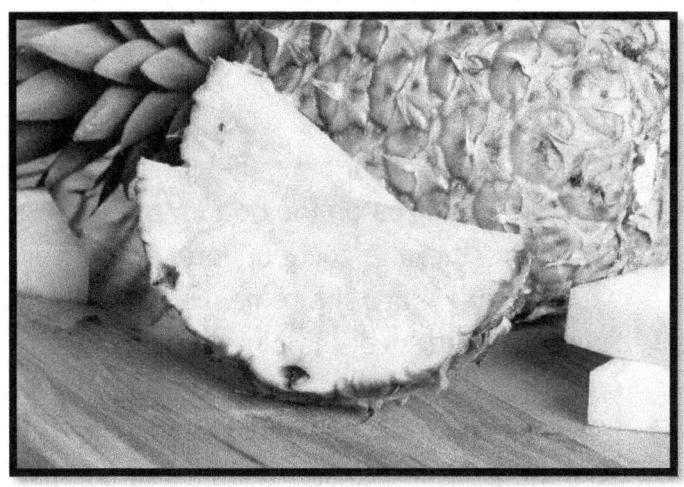

Ingredients:

3 tablespoons coconut oil, divided

5 sliced pineapple rings

¼ cup coconut sugar

1/3 cup sifted coconut flour

5 large eggs, whisked

1 ¼ teaspoon vanilla extract

2 to 3 tablespoons raw honey

¼ cup fresh cherries, pitted and halved

Instructions:

1. Preheat the oven to 350°F and grease a medium cast iron skillet with oil.
2. Heat 2 tablespoons coconut oil in the skillet over medium heat.
3. Place the pineapple rings in the skillet in a single layer and sprinkle with coconut sugar.
4. Cook the mixture for 5 minutes or so until the sugar caramelizes on the bottom of the skillet.
5. Whisk together the coconut flour, eggs, vanilla extract, honey, and the remaining coconut oil.
6. Pour the batter over the pineapple rings and sprinkle with cherries.
7. Place the skillet in the oven and bake for 20 to 25 minutes until a knife inserted in the center comes out clean.
8. Cool the cake completely then turn it out onto a serving dish so the pineapple rings are on top.

Skillet Apple Crisp

Servings: 4

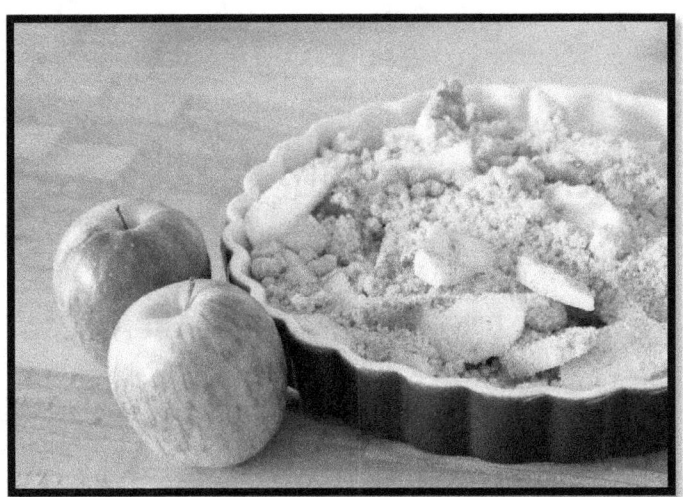

Ingredients:

4 large sweet apples, peeled and sliced thin

1 ¼ teaspoon ground cinnamon

¼ teaspoon ground nutmeg

Pinch salt

1 tablespoon raw honey

½ cup blanched almond flour

2 tablespoons coconut oil, melted

1 tablespoon pure maple syrup

¼ cup chopped walnuts (optional)

Instructions:

1. Preheat the oven to 350°F and lightly grease a medium cast iron skillet.
2. Place the apples in a large mixing bowl and toss with the cinnamon, nutmeg, salt, and honey to coat.
3. Spread the mixture in the skillet and set aside.
4. In a mixing bowl, combine the almond flour, coconut oil, maple syrup, and walnuts.
5. Spread the mixture over the apples and transfer the skillet to the oven.
6. Bake for 50 to 60 minutes until the apples are bubbling and the topping is crisp.

Blueberry Nectarine Cobbler

Servings: 8 to 10

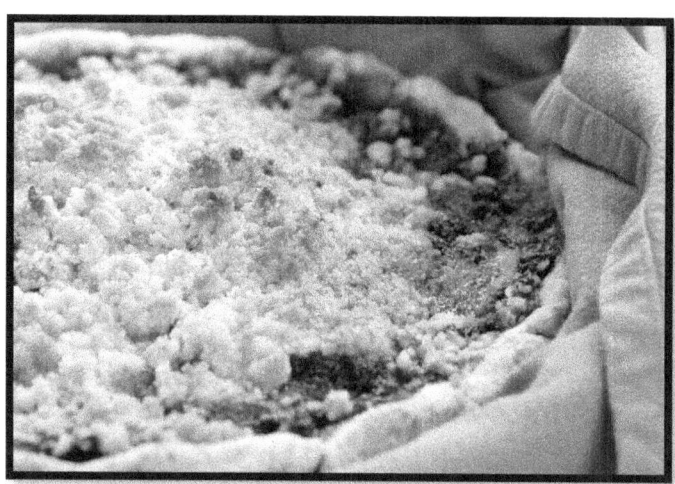

Ingredients:

1/3 cup coconut oil

¾ cup almond flour

2 tablespoons coconut flour

1 ½ teaspoons baking powder

¼ teaspoon salt

1 cup unsweetened almond milk

½ cup coconut sugar

1 teaspoon vanilla extract

2 cups fresh blueberries

3 ripe nectarines, pitted and sliced thin

Instructions:

1. Preheat the oven to 350°F.
2. Place the oil in a large cast iron skillet and put it in the oven for 5 to 6 minutes until the oil is melted.
3. Combine the almond flour, coconut flour, baking powder and salt in a mixing bowl.
4. In a separate bowl, whisk together the almond milk, coconut sugar and vanilla extract.
5. Add the wet ingredients to the dry and whisk until smooth and well combined.
6. Stir the melted coconut oil into the batter and pour it back into the hot skillet.
7. Sprinkle the blueberries and sliced nectarines into the skillet.

8. Bake the cobbler for 45 to 60 minutes until the fruit is bubbling and the batter is set and browned.
9. Cool the cobbler for 15 minutes before serving.

Chocolate Chip Walnut Skillet Cookie

Servings: 12 to 14

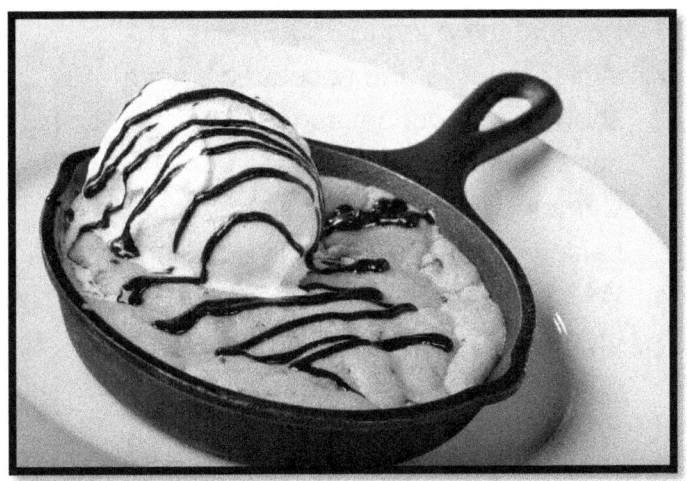

Ingredients:

¾ cup coconut oil

¼ cup palm shortening

1 ¼ cup coconut sugar

¼ cup raw honey

2 cups tapioca flour

½ cup coconut flour

2 teaspoons baking powder

½ teaspoon salt

2 large eggs, beaten

1 cup chopped dark chocolate (at least 65% cacao)

½ cup chopped walnuts

Instructions:

1. Preheat the oven to 350°F.
2. Whisk together the coconut oil, palm shortening, coconut sugar and honey on high speed until it is light and fluffy.
3. Combine the tapioca flour, coconut flour, baking powder, and salt in a mixing bowl.
4. Whisk the egg into the dry ingredients then add the mixture to the wet ingredients and beat until smooth.
5. Fold in the dark chocolate and walnuts.
6. Pour the batter into a large cast iron skillet and place it in the oven.
7. Bake for 22 to 25 minutes until a knife inserted in the center comes out clean.
8. Cool the cookie for 10 minutes then serve with a scoop of coconut milk ice cream.

Conclusion

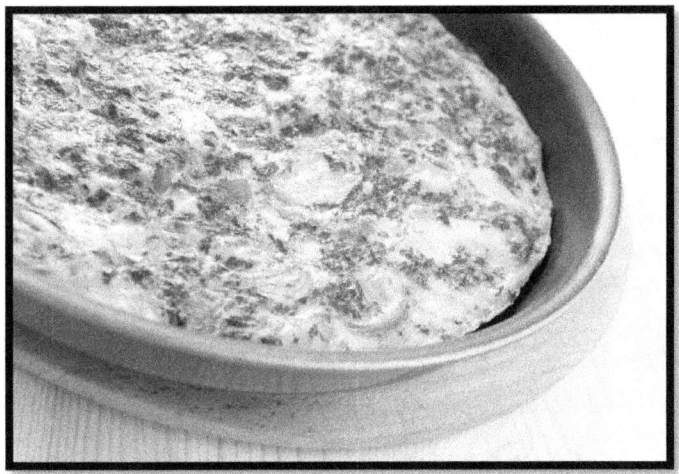

In reading this book, you have learned the basics about the Paleo diet and received a collection of delicious Paleo recipes. Though many people assume that switching to the Paleo diet requires you to give up your favorite foods, this book is proof that you do not. With delicious recipes like Italian Chicken and Mushroom Skillet and Fudgy Chocolate Brownies, you won't even feel like you are on a diet. So what are you waiting for? Try one of these delicious Paleo cast iron skillet recipes today!